The Hair Loss Detective Presents

The Ultimate Guide to

Hair Loss Solutions

Volume Three

By

Leola Anifowoshe, Chief Trichologist

The Author

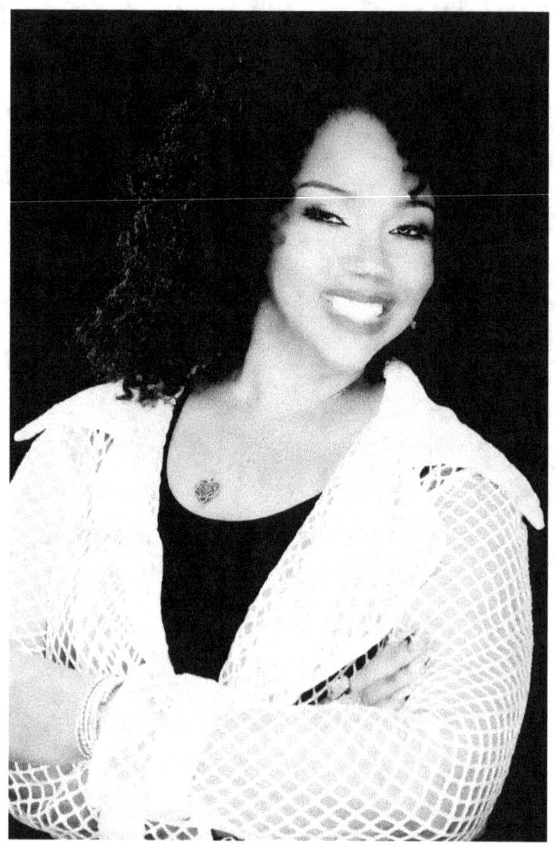

Meet, Chief Trichologist, Leola Anifowoshe, the Founder of Solutions Hair Restoration and Wellness Center. Trichologist Leola has been a hair restoration professional for over 25 years. She keeps her skills modern by attending and hosting hair shows, participating in continuing professional education, and staying closely informed about what's new and effective in the hair restoration and replacement industry.

Ms. Leola is also the Founder of Nzuri Hair Care and Wellness Products. She is passionate about what she does for her patients: how to give people their hair back in the most flattering and undetectable way is always on her mind. As an herbalist and holistic nutrition practitioner sine 1995, Trichologist Leola fully understands the causes of hair loss and offers the right Solution. She has won National awards in hair replacement and also does hair show platform work teaching other cosmetologists her special skill. She is a member of several professional organizations including the National Alopecia Foundation for People of Color, the National Cancer Awareness Committee, The Natural Hair Sorority and the Natural Hair Society.

Through years of extensive training, research and thousand of satisfied clients later, Solutions Hair Restoration has created a multi-therapeutic approach to helping people who suffer from hair loss or slow hair growth problems. "At Solutions, the only goal is to ensure that you leave with a complete solution not a quick fix," says Trichologist Anifowoshe. "When I started in hair care and wellness some 23 years ago I had no idea that my products Nzuri hair growth vitamins and natural hair services would grow to help so many people reclaim their natural born hair back by utilizing our specialized products.

1976 United States Copyright Act, without either the prior written consent of the Publisher.

Disclaimer: The author and publisher have done their best work in preparing the contents of this book, however they make no representations or warranties about the completeness or accuracy of the contents of the book and disclaim any implied warranties of merchantability or fitness for an established or particular purpose. Absolutely no warranty may be created or extended by sales representatives or written sales materials.

The advice and strategies contained in this book may not be suitable for your use. Any use of this content is at your own discretion. You accept full responsibility and liability of any use of this book. The author and publisher shall not be liable for any loss incidental, consequential or other damages of any kind, and will be held completely harmless in all matters.

Anifowoshe, Leola

Hair Loss Solutions Volume One/ by Leola Anifowhoshe

Solutions Hair Restoration Publications

Dedication

This book is dedicated to my loving family that has been with me through my entire journey and my clients that mean the world to me.

Foreword

I am sincerely honored for the invitation to write the Foreword to this absolutely eye-opening book about the mysteries of hair growth and hair loss. What is more, it is not only a source of great pleasure, but also one of total personal gratification to have the privilege of endorsing the work of someone I consider an exceptional person. That is why, in feeling uncommonly blessed to have the rare privilege of celebrating the work of the author, a valued and respected associate of mine, I also consider it an honor to comment on her written work.

The author Leola is a pacesetter, and an entrepreneurial icon in the American Hair Care industry. Those who preach that in every adversity is the seed of an equal and greater benefit may have had this remarkable lady in mind. Although she had developed her awareness of a prodigious interest in beauty, vitamins, health, and wellness quite early in life, it was her later battle with Sarcoidosis that brought her into invaluable knowledge of the overall significance of alternative medicine and nutritional supplements. The rest of her story is simply an incredible story of professionalism and entrepreneurship, as today, she is an acclaimed Master Herbalist, Holistic Therapist and Consultant Trichologist, with eminent specialization in hair loss and repair. In fact, her pedigree in the industry is so unimpeachable that she can be easily called a 'Hair Loss Detective,' solving the mystery of hair loss one strand at a time. Furthermore, her constant research on the physiology of the scalp, and her commitment to the community with reference to the Little Miss "Happy" Head beauty pageants ensures that young girls come into an early and properly-articulated understanding of hair care.

Is the author truly qualified to write a book such as this? My response is an unequivocal "Yes!" After creating Nzuri Elixir, her first and roaringly successful hair product, she went ahead to host her first natural hair show in Houston, Texas, in 2012. Since then, her extraordinarily successful and rapidly evolving brand has introduced in excess of one hundred products that include hair growth shampoos, conditioners and oils. In fact, in my opinion, this book could not be making its debut in a more timely season. I say this because there has never been a more appropriate time in the history of mankind that committed entrepreneurship demands first class professional acumen. It is this unique and original expertise in the art of hair restoration that qualifies the author to be able to write a book that will be of benefit to all stakeholders in the hair care industry.

As a truly alert learner, and a consummate networker and collaborator herself, the author has obviously deployed passion and creativity to hair restoration. Creativity is the active activity of creating something. Because of this, it seems there are many items one will see in the NZURI product line. We must remember that the author had to beat a retreat to the basics, by working with some of the best people in the wellness industry. This led to the creation of her own line of products for NZURI, and as the author herself admits, a compelling issue, Right from the beginning, was to ensure that her ingredients are always of the highest quality, and therefore, as a 100% African American owned and operative hair restoration company, her mission remains the provision of high quality and affordable hair care solutions.

Once more, in my opinion, a subscription to such a high degree of excellence can only lead to equally excellent results. That is why this book is so timely, and so appropriate. And that is why I sincerely commend the book to you. It is a book of simple utility in its delivery of both knowledge and solutions on the distressing subject of hair loss. Additionally, the author has not only presented her work in such a way as to make for infinitely easy reading, assimilation and application, the book is also one finished in exquisite literary taste. Happy reading.

Sam Ennon

BOBSA

President

CEO

Contents

The Science of Hair 1

The Anatomy of Hair and its Follicles 10

Hair Loss Solutions... 12

Nutritional Imbalance 15

Zinc for Hair Loss... 24

Drinking Water and Hair Loss... 30

Different Kinds of Drinking Water....................................... 36

Why A Colon Cleanse?.. 42

Summary 50

Disclaimer 52

Hair Loss Solutions

The Science of Hair

This book will make you an expert on your own hair. After all hair was so important that God had to put it in the bible!

It is a very quick read but highly effective. Remember, it does not have to be complicated to work. It just has to be realistic and work for real. I don't know about you but I am really tired of books that have a lot of fluff and no substance. So I won't do that to you. This short book cuts right to the chase on what helps hair to grow faster. It deals a lot with inside out technology. I know, most books on hair growth deals mostly with topical solutions.

This book will deal with inside out solutions. I cannot guarantee anything except that these Solutions have worked on me, my clients and the thousands of people I've consulted over the years. If you have any health concerns, please consult your Doctor or nutritional advisor. These techniques have been proven safe and effective but every person should always exercise a level of care when it comes to your health and nutrition.

Did you know that within minutes I can know almost everything about you by Looking at Your Hair? The reason is that the hair is so much of a tattle tale of what is going on in your life with your health, sometimes both mentally and physically.

Our hair goes through life's chapters just as we do. I can remember wearing my hair from Blonde to weaves to wigs, to braids and each of those styles somehow depicted where my frame of mind was in those seasons.

I also remember losing all of my hair as a result of prescription drugs. That is what began my journey into healthy hair. So brace yourself as I share with you what I know about hair. Yes, I am a bit more fascinated by hair than most people but perhaps that is because as a Trichologist (A clinically trained hair loss specialist) I know more than most.

I guess I'm obsessed with hair because I've seen the joy it can bring to people as well as the pain. I love sharing information on health and hair. That is why my entire business is dedicated to doing just that. I created the nation's first and only natural hair sorority, Pi Nappa Kappa to empower women around the world to embrace their natural hair. I created the Nzuri Natural Hair & Health Expo (an annual event that has serviced thousands of people over the last several years) to offer educational workshops, fashion shows and products to help consumers "figure out this healthy hair thing". I've created 4 different beauty pageants, Ms. Fab over 40, Ms. Full Figured Foxy, Ms. Top Natural Beauty and even Little Miss Happy Head for the same reasons. "Embrace your natural beauty". And now I am pouring my knowledge out into books for the world to share in my knowledge.

Yes, I Am My Hair. You have to claim it and you have to speak positively about your hair. We all can reckon back to the times when we've spoken poorly about our hair. And as we all should know there is "Power in the Tongue" so ladies, I encourage you to speak life into your hair. If you show me a person with gorgeous hair I will show you a person who speaks positively about their hair. Most women I know who are lifelong weave wearers speak negatively about their hair. So it makes sense why they are confined to the weaves because they've spoken more positively about the weave and has shown much more love and affection about the weaves then their own hair. So try speaking life into your hair, health and relationships and watch the positive changes manifest accordingly.

For a multitude of reasons, your hair may not be growing as fast as you would like it to. Maybe you've noticed your hair starting to thin, or maybe you just want a thicker head of hair. In the following chapters are a variety of easy tips and remedies you can try to help enhance your hair growth, giving you a fuller and healthier look.

This may be the boring part to some of you. But I promise it is good information to know. The biological structure of the hair has been explained to a significant extent by the researchers and according to them, hair is a complicated structure which comprises of the root (or follicle) and the shaft (the visible part of hair). The hair root is enclosed inside the hair follicle, submerges into the skin in inclination and ends down to the bulb.

At the base of hair follicles lie follicular papilla and this structure is very important to the follicle, as it bears capillary vessels which send nutritive elements from blood to hair. In this area are located the receptors and cells that are responsible for hair growth.

The hair shaft is a visible dead part of hair. It consists of 3 layers;

1. **The cuticle** that is built up of colorless, flat overlapping thin scales like cells. It plays a protective role. When the cuticle lies firmly, gently overlapping; hair is silky, soft and shiny. If the cuticle cells are physically or chemically exposed hair loses its shine and becomes brittle and easy to get damaged.

2. The cortex or cortical substance consists of elongated dead cells that give hair strength and elasticity. It also contains the pigment melanin, which determines the natural hair color.

3. The medulla or the ''heart'' of the shaft, which is usually found in the hair of big diameter consists of soft keratin cells and air cavities. The purpose of this layer is unknown, but it is assumed that it transports nutrients to the cortex and the cuticle. This may explain the rapid change of the hair during diseases.

The different layers of the hair shaft are formed by the matrix cells of the bulb. Protein synthesis take place in the matrix cells which contributes to the strength and endurance of the hair shaft. Keratin is a protein that contains sulphur and is being produced in the keratogen zone of the root. Hair consists of proteins (65% - 95%), lipids (1% - 9%), trace elements, polysaccharides and water.

The Anatomy of Hair and its Follicles

The medulla contains melanin pigment granules and is present in only thick terminal hair. It is the least important part of the hair as it pertains to a hair product which nourishes or stimulates hair growth. The cortex, the thickened part of the hair shaft, is a site at which most of the hair changes of texture, porosity, brittleness, color and thickness occurs. The cuticle, consisting of flattened cells arranged like shingles on a roof, maintains the integrity of the hair shaft. The overlapping is extremely tight, preventing damage to the underlying cortex. When the cuticle is intact, the scales are smooth, reflect light, and provide the hair with a shiny, healthy look. This healthy appearance is a manifestation of the hair's porosity, elasticity, and texture.

Vitamins and Hair Loss

Our hair requires some essential vitamins for healthy growth, should you be suffering from hair fall the use of vitamins for hair loss will provide all the required ingredients. The majority of these vitamins should include B complex vitamins, Inositol, and Vitamins A and E.

Vitamins are necessary for your body's health as well as your hair health. But the truth of the matter is that most vitamin products are ineffective and even the best selling brands contain toxins. Indeed taking vitamin supplements will benefit your health but only if taken correctly.

Many of these vitamins assist in hair growth and make them healthy and strong. While others nourish the scalp strengthening each hair strand and giving the overall healthy shiny finish. Hair loss vitamins including 4-aminobenzoic acid help your hair by preventing them from turning grey.

These vitamins for hair loss may not be able to help you grow hair back naturally in case the follicles of your hair are already damaged. The use of vitamins on their own is not enough to repair damaged follicles. They possibly will help the remaining hair to be healthier, stronger and grow faster but they cannot help you grow hair back from the hair follicles that are already dead.

Hair loss is down to a number of contributing factors not just genetics, poor diets and stress are among the top ones. An improper diet does not supply the sufficient amount of nutrients required by the body to function normally. Any deficiency or nutrient shortage in the body is reflected by the unhealthy hair.

Nutritional Imbalance

One of the most common causes of hair loss is an insufficiency of one or more vitamins and minerals in the body. **This is my primary reason for developing vitamins specifically for hair growth**. We'll talk more about vitamins and minerals that contribute to the proper functioning of the hair follicles, qualitative blood circulation of the scalp and growth of hair.

The most important vitamins that affect the health of the hair include vitamins A and E, almost the entire group of B vitamins, iron, zinc, calcium, selenium and others. The most acute hair suffers from a lack of vitamins of group B. This vitamin is responsible for the proper metabolism, pigmentation and hair growth process.

Thiamine (B1) provides carbohydrate and fat metabolism in the body and participates in an oxygen inflow to the follicles, while

Riboflavin (B2) helps to correct its flow. This vitamin is also involved in redox reactions in the blood supply to the follicles.

Lack of nicotinic acid (Vitamin PP) can lead to disturbed oxidative processes in the body, loss of pigmentation (appearance of early gray hair), breakage and hair loss.

Pantothenic acid (B5) impacts on the supply of hair follicles with oxygen and regulating their growth, strength and development.

Pyridoxine (Vit. B6) deficiency leads to abnormalities in amino acid production which may result in dry skin, dandruff and hair loss.

Inositol (Vitamin B8) promotes active absorption of other vitamins of its group and vitamin E, while

Folic acid (B9) has a positive effect on cell division throughout the body and promotes hair growth.

Niacin (Vitamin B3)

Niacin has the ability to dilate blood vessels. This may help hair growth by ensuring the capillaries in the scalp are flushed and capable of delivering nutrients to the hair follicles. Foods rich in niacin include fish, red meat, celery, dairy, beans, almonds, and carrots.

The most popular vitamin which is known as Biotin helps supplying nutrition to scalp and the tone of the hair, providing the natural pigmentation of the hair.

The lack of cobalamin (vitamin B12) may lead to patchy hair loss. **All of these vitamins are scientifically blended into the Nzuri Hair Vitamins Liquid or Capsules. (More about this later).**

Other vitamins that prevent hair loss are Vitamin A, E and C. Vitamin A helps the hair to protect their elasticity and strength over the entire length; Vitamin E is responsible for a good blood flow of the scalp, hair pigmentation and regulation of the immune system and Vitamin C helps iron absorption, stimulates hair growth and protects the hair follicles from destruction.

One particular vitamin that can be of assistance is vitamin E. A vital vitamin for encouraging blood circulation in the scalp will insure the right nutrients get to the follicles for better growth. Vitamins E can be found in most leafy green vegetables. The downside to this is that people not eating enough vegetables will not obtain the required amounts of vitamins needed.

It's surprising to know that many people forget that a healthy body needs a healthy diet and this will reflect in healthy hair. When you reach a desperate state of hair loss searching for a miracle cure is the first thing everyone looks for, but many a time the core of the problem is in the foods you eat.

Apart from vitamin E and all the vitamins mentioned earlier, fatty acids are another essential dietary requirement. Canola oil, walnuts, soy and fish should be consumed, as they are rich in fatty acids. It is suggested by research that intakes of omega-3 fatty acids and fish are connected to reduced rates of depression. Since stress and depression lead to hair loss upping your intake of omega-3 will reduce the risk of depression.

Taking vitamins to grow hair back cannot be of help until and unless you have a proper and healthy diet. Finding a good source of nutritonal foods full of the requirements for hair loss will help prevent further problems and possibly reverse some damage if caught in time.

Moreover, the cause of hair loss can also be due to a lack of trace elements in the body. Some of these elements are responsible for a better circulation and nutrition of the hair.

Iron is an essential mineral for healthy hair. Its deficiency leads to slower processes in the body and impaired oxygen metabolism. Iron deficiency often causes split ends, fragile hair and baldness in women. Iron deficiency, today is the most common cause of hair loss in girls of childbearing age. While iron can be achieved by food and supplement, we should not forget that Vitamin C contributes to a better absorption of iron.

Next on the list is Zinc. Zinc is a mineral that is responsible for the regulation of male sex hormones and it also affect the health and integrity of the hair. It is also believed that Zinc deficiency can cause dryness of the scalp. Zinc deficiency is also linked with a condition known as "alopecia" (hair loss). Thus, Zinc plays an important role in regulating the sebaceous glands of the scalp and normal hair growth.

Intake of sulphur involved in collagen formation or the formation of "building blocks" of the hair, while Calcium deficiency is also a cause of disastrous consequences like poor quality of hair and hair loss.

Selenium is involved in the "transport" of the materials necessary for hair growth and Magnesium deficiency leads to intensive hair loss, dryness and brittleness. Among all of these necessary vitamins and minerals iodine cannot be missed in any case. **All of** these vitamins and minerals are scientifically blended into the Nzuri Hair Vitamins Liquid or Capsules.

Zinc for Hair Loss

There are many reasons why we need zinc in our bodies. These reasons include:

- Aiding in the absorption of other nutrients

- Building healthy cells

- Regulating hormones

Zinc helps to keep hormone levels regulated, which is one of the reasons why it is so effective in preventing and treating hair loss.

The Zinc Balance

Just as zinc deficiency can cause hair loss, so can excess zinc. A high level of zinc in the body not only disrupts the absorption of other essential minerals such as magnesium and iron, it also promotes the production of testosterone.

High testosterone levels coupled with other hormonal imbalances lead to hair thinning and eventually hair loss. On the other hand, iron deficiency is an identified cause of hair loss.

Therefore, just as zinc deficiency causes loss of hair through multiple paths so does excess zinc in the body. In a way, this is good news since it means that zinc is very important to the growth of hair follicles.

High doses of zinc are reported to inhibit both the anagen and catagen stages of hair growth.

How Zinc Prevents Hair Loss

To understand how zinc prevents hair loss, it is important to know how zinc deficiency can lead to hair loss.

One theory established that zinc deficiency leads to changes in the protein structure of hair follicles leading to weakening of their structural integrity. This means new hairs will fall off quicker than they should. The importance of zinc to hair regrowth has been confirmed in lab rats.

Furthermore, there are recorded cases of people whose hair changed back from dull, aging gray to their original colors when placed on diets rich in zinc. Another study puts the importance of zinc to hair regrowth on the mineral's crucial role in DNA and RNA production. This is a requirement for the efficient division of follicle cells leading to an improved anagen (growth) stage of the hair growth cycle.

In addition, the effectiveness of zinc in reversing hair loss due to negative enzymatic reactions has been demonstrated in topical application of the mineral.

The recommended daily intake of zinc is 8 – 11 mg but the recommended daily dose of the mineral is 15 mg delivered as a chelate. While the recommended doses are put on the safe side of treatment, some hair loss experts advocate an upper limit of 25 mg.

However, to prevent excessive zinc intake, zinc supplementation should not be taken at this upper limit for longer than 2 – 3 weeks.

Since zinc reduces the amount of copper in the body, the recommendation is to take a little copper supplement alongside.

Also, zinc supplementation is often paired with selenium supplementation because the latter is a known antioxidant which protects pathways known to promote hair growth.

On the other hand, zinc reduces the absorption of calcium and vice versa. For this reason, Zinc supplements formulated with calcium should be avoided. Similarly, zinc should not be taken with foods such as milk or cheese with high calcium content. You won't have to worry about these combinations with any Nzuri supplements as we have already taken precautions to ensure that they are formulated properly.

It should not be taken alongside fibrous food too since dietary fiber binds minerals and prevent their absorption. Lean meat, on the other hand, as well as shellfish, fish and eggs improve the absorption of zinc.

Drinking Water and Hair Loss

Something that is often overlooked is the effect of water and dehydration on hair loss. Each hair shaft is 1/4 water and when you don't drink enough, it causes your hair to become weak. Water also helps to flush your body of toxins which could be a major contributor to hair loss.

Water is a natural miracle ingredient which supports <u>hair vitamin</u> consumption while assisting in healthy and efficient hair growth.

Did I say water? Yes indeed. If you're going to make the emotional, mental, financial and long term commitment to take hair growth vitamins, it's important you also be prepared to crank up your daily water consumption.

Water is essential for proper hair growth. Be sure to get plenty of that H2O for growing healthy hair that is soft, supple and lush.

Water makes up approximately one fourth of the weight of a strand of hair and when hair has the proper amount of water, it will respond by being supple, and shiny.

Drink a minimum of 8 to 10 glasses (8 ounce serving) of water a day to get gleaming healthy tresses.

Hair Dehydration

There are other factors in hair dehydration. The surface skin which composes the human scalp that houses hair roots is made up of a thicker tissue than the interior tissues of the body.

Circulation flows to the base of the skin which covers the scalp and the hair roots. Water has to seep upwards through all the layers of the skin to reach the outer layers.

Hair must receive adequate water through its roots or the supply will fall short of reaching budding layers.

The exposed surface of hair roots are constantly losing water due to environmental factors such as sun, wind, hard water, and chemicals. In essence this natural water loss creates a type of double jeopardy.

When the body is dehydrated, circulation to the base of the outer skin, the scalp and hair roots, may be shut down as an emergency measure by the body's drought management system.

The drought management system works to make sure water is not lost through evaporation from the skin's surface.

Water and Hydration

You may have heard how drinking lots of water can help keep your skin hydrated and looking younger. Hair is actually a connective tissue of the body and carries many of the same compositions as your skin, fingernails and toenails. When you don't get enough water into your system, the result is dehydration, and for many, hair loss as well. As a matter of fact, **75% of the population is dehydrated and not even aware of it!**

Some of the signs of mild dehydration are as follows:

Feeling tired	Signs of severe dehydration are as follows:
Feeling thirsty	Extreme thirst
Decreased urine output. If you have not been to the bathroom in eight hours, you are most likely dehydrated.	No tears when crying
	Irritability
	Confusion
	Little or no urination
Dry skin	Sunken eyes
Headaches	Low blood pressure
Constipation	Fever
	Rapid heartbeat
Feeling dizzy or light headed	Dry skin that does not bounce back when pinched
Thirst	Very dry mouth

Different Kinds of Drinking Water

Not all water is the same! The best kind of water to drink is natural spring water. It's natural, wholesome and as real as it can get. For those of you that drink bottled water, natural spring water should be your first choice as it provides the best hydration for your hair and body.

Another good choice is steam distilled water. One that should be avoided is purified water. Why? Because purified water (reverse osmosis water) does not hydrate your hair and body well at all. Some other types of drinking water that contains reverse osmosis water include Dasani and Aqua Fina as well as most sparkling waters.

Distilled water should not be consumed for more than just a few months because it does not have the minerals that natural spring water has and will eventually start to leach these minerals from your body. If you prefer to drink tap water, it should be carbon filtered.

It is important to drink enough water. The average adult should be drinking at least three quarts of water every day and even more when it is hot outside or if you are physically active.

Parasites

There are a number of reasons for hair loss and hair shedding. One that is often overlooked is parasites. Poor nutrition can occur when parasites steal nutrients from the body. Parasites create acidity in the body. They produce toxic waste and rob nutrients. The Nzuri Parasite Flush Out program includes herbs that have anti-bacterial abilities which kill the harmful parasites.

Millions of people in the U.S. may be suffering from health problems caused by a condition of which they are completely unaware. The problems are caused by parasites--something which is usually associated with people living in third world countries. A study published in "The American Journal of Tropical Medicine and Hygiene" revealed that 32% of a nationally representative sample of 2,896 people tested positive for parasites.

One symptom is the affect of parasites on the organs in the body. Because parasites emit toxins that can over work the liver and kidneys, the organs may become sluggish leading to weight gain, fatigue and irritability. Certain herbs have been shown to kill parasites in the body helping to reverse their ill effects. Nzuri Parasite Flush Out includes these key herbs and other important nutrients in a formulation that is one of the strongest available.

Nzuri Parasite Flush Out helps cleanse and release a variety of parasitic organisms. Helps normalize digestive tract processes to prevent re-infestation.*

This is a combination herbal remedy formula containing a powerful blend of active herbs to help rid the body of parasites. Several types of parasites can live inside human intestines, blood, the lymphatic system, bile ducts, or organs, such as the liver. Nzuri Parasite Flush Out attacks parasites at their attachments, allowing the body the ability to actively remove the invaders. Parasite diseases are not some 'way out there' illness. In fact, studies have shown that 1 in 3 people have parasites.

They have become such a common problem even the CDC (Center for Disease Control) website, lists 'Parasite Diseases' as one of the selections under their category 'Diseases and Conditions'. There are a number of reasons for hair loss and hair shedding. One that is often overlooked is parasites. Poor nutrition can occur when parasites steal nutrients from the body. Parasites create acidity in the body. They produce toxic waste and rob nutrients.

The Nzuri Parasite Flush out program includes herbs that have anti-bacterial abilities that kill the harmful parasites. An impacted colon, parasites, metals and hidden infections contribute to poor assimilation of nutrients that feed the hair. Parasite cleansing is the process of killing these harmful organisms living inside your bodies and flushing them out. These herbs are not harmful to us and if you make it part of your routine to take them regularly, it can rid your whole digestive tract of parasites.

Why A Colon Cleanse?

We live in a stress filled environment. Filled with unavoidable toxins, such as the water we drink the food we eat and the air that we breathe. Toxins are present in pharmaceutical drugs, metals, hormones and chemicals.

Your body has seven elimination channels which remove these toxins, efficiently when your system isn't overburdened. However, when these channels become overburdened we lose the ability to properly eliminate these health and beauty robbers. Essentially, the colon stops functioning properly.

Once the colon stops functioning properly to eliminate waste, disease will easily come into our bodies. Beauty and health destroying diseases such as cancer, autoimmune disorders, dull lifeless hair and skin, and a host of other conditions we don't want, can and will creep into our bodies.

Many of us do not have the necessary 1 to 3 bowel movements per day. It is not uncommon for someone to have 5+ pounds of fecal matter backed up in their colon. Can you imagine that? It's a very scary thought indeed. It's not uncommon for the average person to have only 1 to 2 bowel movements a week!

This is the perfect environment for toxins to thrive in your body. Those who have done colon cleanses often discover a renewed feeling of rejuvenation, they are often more alert, lose weight, notice improvements in hair and skin conditions. Many even report improvement with depression and anxiety - two hair and skin robbing conditions. And the improved digestion will help with the absorption of the necessary nutrients your body needs to be healthy and beautiful.

Here Is the Key – Quality! It is very important to note that there are A LOT of colon cleanses available. Since natural health supplements are not regulated, it is important that you purchase from a reputable company. Always research the product before purchasing. If reviews are available that's all the better.

There are other reputable cleanses on the market, but I like to stick with what I know works. Nzuri Kra-Z Hair Gro Hair Booster 15 Day Colon Cleanse works wonders. Nzuri understands hair growth and we understand internal consumption of hair supplements.

The 15-Day Cleanse formula will provide results within 12 to 24 hours in terms of helping rid the intestinal tract of excess waste, reduce bloating, help increase energy and may provide several pounds of weight loss within a few days. Included in the formula are effective natural laxatives, fiber, herbs which help soothe the intestinal lining and Acidophilus to help promote healthy bacteria levels in the intestinal tract. While this product may not be used on a daily basis beyond the 15-day cleanse period, it may be used occasionally for intestinal cleaning with the 15-day cleanse repeated several weeks following the initial cleanse.

Nzuri 15 Day Colon Cleanse

The colon is so important that some experts have labeled it the 2nd brain. Nzuri's Hair Booster 15-Day Cleanse works wonders to prepare your body to receive all the necessary vitamins and nutrients it needs to thrive at its full capacity. Toxemia (systemic poisoning) is the most pervasive condition that plagues our modern civilization. Never before in the history of mankind have our bodies been exposed to such a vast array of toxic substances from our food supply, the air we breathe, the water we drink and use to bathe, and electromagnetic pollution. The effects these poisons have on the body can be observed in the rampant and growing number of degenerative and autoimmune diseases. The incidence of cancer (especially colo-rectal, breast, and prostate) and the number of individuals suffering from allergies has reached an all-time high.

Nzuri Vida 10 in 1 Stress and Energy Tonic.

What does energy have to do with hair growth or hair loss you ask? It has a lot to do with it. When is the last time you were able to operate at maximum efficiency on low energy? You were not. And neither are your hair follicles. Also, since stress is the number one cause of hair loss, we've added essential ingredients in this product to help lower the endorphins that causes your body to react to stress.

This product is also loaded with antioxidants that help to kill free radicals. Free radicals are invaders. They're like gang members and bullies. They wreak havoc on our system. Antioxidants are like law enforcement. They keep peace and order in a disorderly environment. You wouldn't want to be in a gang infested area without law enforcement would you? So why put your insides to the test of no protection from the bullies Free radicals? Yes, radical they are.

They cause oxidation (cell degeneration) and left unchecked they will have more than your hair falling out.   This is another reason eating organic berries and fruits are good. They are loaded with antioxidants. NzuriVida 10 in 1 Stress and Energy Tonic is made with 3 very effective, anti-oxidant rich fruits from the Amazon rainforest. They are acai berry, cupucua (coo-pwa-soo) and yerba mate which is a higher level of green tea. So no guess work on why this phyto nutrient rich powerhouse does the cells good and you feel it in 15 minutes!

Summary

The bottom line is that you have to have a system for healthy hair in order to make your hair grow and grow faster. No matter what anyone says, as long as there is life there is hope. Your hair can grow.

1. You need to be able to do scalp massages,

2. Take Nzuri Hair Vitamins daily

3. Eat more fruits and vegetables.

4. Get together a hair journal. Put down your favorite products and why. We sometimes forget what they are so that is why a hair journal is good until it becomes a routine.

5. Take it easy and be patient. The only thing that can really help hair grow longer is time.

6. Use protective styling. Too much manipulation can cause hair to fall out.

Disclaimer

I am not a medical doctor. I am clinically trained in Trichology. A **'Trichologist'** is someone who specializes in hair loss problems such as baldness, hair breakage and itchy/flaking scalp. He or she will also treat all forms of alopecia.

This book is not intended as a substitute for the medical advice of physicians. The reader should regularly consult a physician in matters relating to his/her health and particularly with respect to any symptoms that may require diagnosis or medical attention.

No part of this book may be reproduced without express written permission from the author. If you want to use part of this book, get permission or use Written by Trichologist Leola Anifowoshe.

If you have any healthy problems or are in doubt consult your doctor or nutritionist to know the exact intake that you need to have.

For speaking engagements, contact us at

Solutionshairrestore@gmail.com

Visit our website: www.TexasHairLossClinic.com

Get all of your healthy hair care products here:

www.HairVitaminStore.com